ANAHATA

CHAKRA
Awakening & Healing

Shreyanada Natha

Cover & Design
Mattias Långström

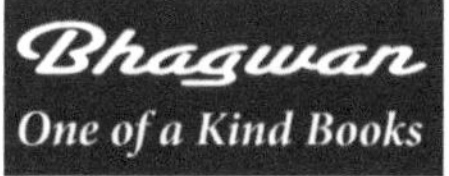

Bhagwan
One of a Kind Books

ANAHATA
CHAKRA
Awakening & Healing

Shreyanada Natha

ISBN 9789198915457

✷✷✷

BHAGWAN 2024

1 FREE BONUS!

#1. *Download* **CHAKRA-INDEX IN COLOR** *here!*

SCAN QR-CODE or go to:

https://bit.ly/47wdFVZ

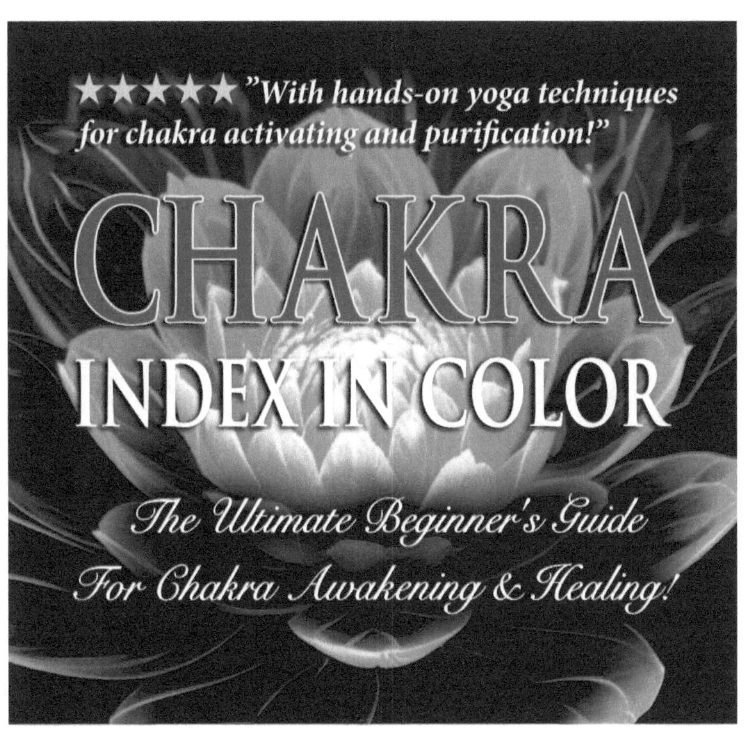

ABOUT THE BOOK:

Kickstart your spiritual awakening! Wonderful yogic deep relaxation and meditation with unique Anahata chakra awakening and healing. Including authentic Anahata Yoga Nidra script!

PRESENTATION

Yoga Nidra, or yogic sleep, is a unique meditation process that`s powerfully profound and healing for body, mind, and spirit. Practitioners are led into a state of deep relaxation and the experience of our chakra system.

Yoga Nidra offers extensive benefits, yet it is one of the most straightforward yoga practices. All you have to do is put on your most comfortable clothes, find a quiet space, lie down on your back, and listen to the meditation. The book includes an authentic Manipura Yoga Nidra script!

MY NAME AND MY MISSION

Shreyananda Natha was the name I received when I was initiated into the Natha Order and received the master mantra—Shodasi-mantra—after studying yoga and tantra for over twelve years. Shodasi-mantra is the highest mantra in yoga and tantra. It means "he who knows."

After practicing yoga and meditation continuously for over 20 years, having a yoga school for many years, and leading studies for yoga teachers, I wanted to reach out more broadly with yoga, out into our whole society, out of the little yoga room. Spread the knowledge of yoga, our chakra system, and Kundalini Shakti to everyone who wants to listen. What needed to be added were sensible factual books on yoga that were in-depth educational and not just skim the surface or were about the author's private life. So it became my Sankalpa, my magical wish, and my mission to create exciting yoga books that everyone can read and enjoy. To show how we can apply and use yoga in different parts of life and achieve success and health. Here and now. So, if you like my books, please follow me on my social media, share and like them, tell your friends about them, and write an honest review; one or two lines don't matter. All support is precious.

MY YOUTUBE CHANNEL

*My YouTube channel, **YOGA BEYOND THE POSES**, has been a significant project for me. I wanted to create a channel containing my two most extensive life interests: yoga, of course, and everything related to the mystery of life, the spiritual and the psychic. Yes, everything related to the expansion of our consciousness. What we experience in yoga beyond the poses...*

I broadcast LIVE on YouTube, and during the broadcast, I talk about yoga and spirituality and let viewers ask questions that I answer with the help of runes and what I receive as a medium. It's completely free, and it would be great to hear your question and see what the runes say about it. You can sub-scribe to the channel to quickly get notifications before each broadcast so you don't miss any exciting questions.

Scan the QR code or visit:

https://shorturl.at/dqx36

THE AUTHOR

Shreyananda Natha is the author of popular and best-selling yoga books. He has written one of the most comprehensive books on yoga – EVERYTHING ABOUT YOGA and the study book – TEACHING YOGA AND MEDITATION BEYOND THE PO-SES. He is also a certified yoga & meditation teacher according to the international guidelines of EYTF. He has undergone several years of yoga teacher training under the guidance of Swami Omananda at Satyananda Ashram and holds the highest initiation in the tantric Natha order. He frequently travels to Asia and India to deepen his knowledge and gather inspiration. He has immersed himself in tantric rituals and is known for his extensive knowledge of yoga, deep relaxation, and meditation.

"There is no authority that can say what yoga is. When you give yourself completely and thoroughly and experience yoga without limitations and doubts, the actual meeting with yoga arises when you become one with the experience within you. Only then do you understand what yoga is – for you. When you are no longer limited by modesty, shyness, and artificial thought patterns that act as a filter between you and trans-formation.

Yoga is a cultural richness still passed on from teacher to student and helps man find his true nature. It opens us up and attracts awareness. It strengthens our self-esteem, and our entire spectrum of possibilities suddenly becomes visible. Yoga is easy and normal. You don't need to become vegan, a monk, or be able to stand on your head. You need to do your yoga regularly; the rest will come naturally. You can use yoga and meditation to feel better physically and mentally and succeed and develop in all areas of life – here and now.

Good luck!"

NAMASTÉ

I want to thank the teachers and students I have had over the years who have made my journey with yoga so enjoyable. Thank you for all the inspiration you have given me and for making this book possible. The yoga masters who no longer live among us – live on with each new person who delves into the yoga tradition.

Sri Swami Sivananda, Sri Swami Satyananda, Sri Tirumalai Krishnamacharya, Sri Swami Vishnudevananda, Sri K. Pattabhi Jois, Osho, Swami Nirdosha, Swami Omananda, Swami Janakananda, Ole Schmidt, Turiya, Maryam Abrishami, and Sanna Kuittinen.

All the people who have sought answers to what they have sensed through an activated Ajna chakra. In yoga, they have learned the principles behind the universe, the collective consciousness, and the creative power, Kundalini Shakti. The duality behind everything, both what we see and what we don't see. Together, we help pass on the previously secret knowledge about our gunas, nadis, and chakras to everyone who wants to be a Rishi.

Aum Shri Durgayai Namaha

1

RELAXATION & MEDITATION

Meditation has long been known for its positive effects on health and well-being, and research has increasingly confirmed its many benefits. By reducing stress and promoting inner calm, meditation can be a powerful resource for improving physical and mental health.

A study published in the journal "JAMA Internal Medicine" found that mindfulness meditation reduced levels of the stress hormone cortisol in participants, resulting in improved feelings of well-being and reduced experience of stress.

Research has also shown that meditation can positively affect the brain and cognitive functions. A meta-analysis published in the journal "Neuroscience & Biobehavioral Reviews" found that meditation can increase gray matter volume in the brain, linked to improved cognitive function and reduced age-related decline in brain tissue.

Meditation has also been shown to have beneficial effects on the physical level. A review article published in the journal

Annals of the New York Academy of Sciences summarized research showing that meditation can lower blood pressure, reduce inflammation, and improve immune system function.

In addition to its physical and mental health benefits, meditation can also promote emotional balance and increase emotional intelligence. A study published in the journal *Psychological Science* found that regular meditation increased participants' ability to manage negative emotions and emotional stability.

In summary, research has clearly shown that meditation can positively affect health and well-being. By reducing stress, improving cognitive functions, promoting emotional balance, and supporting physical health, meditation can be a powerful resource for promoting an overall healthy lifestyle and increasing quality of life.

REFERENCES

Rosenkranz, M. A., Davidson, R. J., Maccoon, D. G., Sheridan, J. F., Kalin, N. H., & Lutz, A. (2013). A comparison of mindfulness-based stress reduction and an active control in modulation of neurogenic inflammation. Brain, Behavior, and Immunity, 27(1), 174-184.

Fox, K. C., Nijeboer, S., Dixon, M. L., Floman, J. L., Ellamil, M., Rumak, S. P., ... & Christoff, K. (2014). Is meditation associated with altered brain structure? A systematic review and meta-analysis of morphometric neuroimaging in meditation practitioners. Neuroscience & Biobehavioral Reviews, 43, 48-73.

Pascoe, M. C., Thompson, D. R., Jenkins, Z. M., & Ski, C. F. (2017). Mindfulness mediates the physiological markers of stress: Systematic review and meta-analysis. Journal of Psychiatric Research, 95, 156-178.

Desbordes, G., Negi, L. T., Pace, T. W., Wallace, B. A., Raison, C. L., & Schwartz, E. L. (2012). Effects of mindful-attention and compassion meditation training on amygdala response to emotional stimuli in an ordinary, non-meditative state. Frontiers in Human Neuroscience, 6, 292.

2

ANAHATA CHAKRA AWAKENING & HEALING

Authentic Yoga Nidra Meditation Script

ANAHATA CHAKRA AWAKENING & HEALING

Authentic Yoga Nidra Meditation Script.

Yogic deep relaxation/meditation – Introduction.

Yoga Nidra, also known as yogic sleep, is a unique meditation practice that is deeply powerful and healing for the body, mind, and soul. It has its roots in the oldest Indian and tantric scriptures. It was originally developed from the tantric nyasa techniques, which were used to incorporate and vitalize the body and mind with universal energy. Specific mantras are placed on various parts of the body to activate energy centers and release blockages along the subtle energy channel known as nadis and energy centers known as chakras.

According to tantric traditions, the foundation of nyasa techniques lies in achieving a deeper awareness of the body and energy flow and attaining a profound spiritual understanding and experience. By focusing the mind on different body parts and visualizing specific mantras or sounds, the practitioner can create a strong connection between body, mind, and spirit and achieve a sense of inner balance and harmony.

Yoga Nidra, which evolved from these nyasa techniques, is a form of guided meditation and relaxation where practitioners are guided through a series of steps to achieve deep relaxation and awareness. During a typical Yoga Nidra session, participants are led through a systematic relaxation exercise that includes body awareness, breathing exercises, visualizations, and affirmations to promote deep relaxation and inner stillness.

The benefits of Yoga Nidra include reduced stress and anxiety, improved sleep quality, increased body awareness and relaxation, and promoting inner peace and well-being. Through regular practice of Yoga Nidra, the practitioner can experience a sense of deep inner calm and peace as well as increased clarity and concentration.

The original nyasa techniques and their philosophy and practice can be found in several classic tantric texts, including Tantrasara, Vijnanabhairava Tantra, and Shiva Svarodaya. These texts offer insights and guidance on practicing nyasa to enhance the mind and experience more profound awareness and spirituality. Exploring these texts with the help of authorized teachers and guides can be a way to understand and appreciate the rich tradition of Nyasa and its role in the development of Yoga Nidra and other meditation techniques.

Yoga Nidra offers comprehensive benefits but is one of the most straightforward yoga practices. All you need to do is put on your most comfortable clothes, find a quiet space, sit on a comfy chair, or lie on your back and listen to the meditation.

INSTRUCTIONS

Your sankalpa (your decision and desire) should never be revealed to anyone. Doing so diminishes its power.

YOGA NIDRA – ANAHATA CHAKRA AWAKENING & HEALING. CA 60 MIN

YOU INTRODUCE

Get ready for yoga nidra ... lie down in shavasana and straighten your clothes, so you lie comfortably and feel no need to move. 1 MIN

GENTLE START

Get ready for yoga nidra ... 1 MIN

Lie down in the shavasana and straighten your clothes, so you lie comfortably and do feel the need to move again. 1 MIN

Now, concentrate on the body. 1 MIN

Become aware of the silence of the body. 1 MIN

You lie completely still as if your body were made of stone. 1 MIN

Aware of the body – body awareness. 1 MIN

Listen to all the sounds around you. 1 MIN

All sounds simultaneously, effortlessly. 1MIN

Tell yourself ... I'm awake and going to practice yoga nidra, I'm not going to fall asleep. 1 MIN

Now it's time to make your Sankalpa. Your inner wish. Your decision for this yoga nidra ... 1 MIN

Positive, clear and distinct – 3 times, you say it quietly to yourself.

It goes deep into your subconscious and is bound to manifest. 3MIN

Repeat the body parts after me in your head and fill them with your consciousness – go to your right hand ... 1 MIN

Thumb on your right side, index finger, middle finger, ring finger, little finger, hand, arm, shoulder, armpit, chest, abdomen, thigh, knee, shin, foot, big toe, second toe, third toe, fourth toe and so little toe, feel the whole of your right side ... 2 MIN

Take your consciousness to your left side ... feel your left thumb, index finger, middle finger, ring finger, little finger, hand, arm, shoulder, armpit, chest, abdomen, thigh, knee, shin, foot, big toe, second toe, third toe, fourth toe and so little toe, feel the whole of your left side ... 2 MIN

Feel the back of your head, neck, shoulders, spine, entire back ... buttocks, thighs, back knees, calves, feet ... feel the entire back of your whole body ... 2 MIN

Feel the top of the head, forehead, nose, tip of the nose, lips, chin tip, neck, collarbone, chest, arms, navel, inside the navel, genitals, thighs, knees, shins, feet, toes ... 2 MIN

Feel the whole right arm, the whole left arm, the whole right leg, left leg, torso, head ... the whole body ... 2 MIN

Concentrate now on breathing ... experience it, do not control it ... go to the left nostril, feel how you draw in air and how it goes out through the right nostril ... feel the temperature difference at the upper lip ... 1 MIN

On 1 you draw in air through the left nostril, on 1 out through the right, on 2 in through the right and 2 out through the left ... on 5, 10, 15 etc. you draw in air through both nostrils and out through both. Count carefully, if you count incorrectly, start again from 1 ... 10 MIN

Anahata chakra awakening ... I MIN

*Go to Anahata chakra in the center of the chest ... feel the pul-
sation there and say quietly to yourself ... YAM 3 times ...
1 MIN*

*See Anahata chakra in front of your close eyes in chidakasha
... in microcosm ... see a a blue lotus with twelve petals, see the
lotus clearly to your inner self ... 3 MIN*

*See the following objects in front of you, touch them, smell
them ...*

a desert, 1 MIN

pyramid, 1 MIN

temple, 1 MIN

a Buddha statue, 1 MIN

a rose, 1 MIN

waves far out to sea, 1 MIN

candle flame, 1 MIN

sunrise, 1 MIN

birds flying, 1 MIN

clouds, 1 MIN

yin and yang, 1 MIN

Shiva, 1 MIN

a triangle with the tip down, 1 MIN

a triangle with the tip up, 1 MIN

triangels lying on top of each other so they form a six-pointed star, 1 MIN

a circle, 1 MIN

a square, 1 MIN

experience happiness, 1 MIN

a golden egg, 1 MIN

a pulsating white glow at the center of the eyebrows ... 1 MIN a daisy lotus flower on top of your head … 1 MIN

Now it's time to repeat your decision, your sankalpa – clearly,
3 times …

I say Hari Om Tat Sat 3 times and then yoga nidra is over for
this time
3 MIN

ENDING
Hari Om Tat Sat 3 times. 1 MIN

… we can now open our eyes and start moving our bodies … 3
MIN

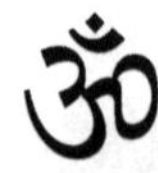

Did you like the book? Feel free to follow me on my social media, share and like, tell your friends about the books, and feel free to write an honest review; one or two lines don't matter. All support is precious. Thanks!

On my Facebook page and Instagram, I post exciting news and tips on temporary offers and benefits you can take advantage of. I often also post my yoga routine and other things related to nutrition and health that may be interesting to take part in. So feel free to join them so you don't miss anything interesting:

 *facebook.com/bhagwanoneofakindbooks*

 *instagram.com/bhagwanoneofakindbooks/*

MY BOOKS AND BOOK SERIES

I have two book series that have different audiences. Great Yoga Books – is a series with the most comprehensive fact books on yoga for those who want to explore the subject in depth. Here, you will also find classic yoga books that are rarely translated, such as Patanjali's Yoga Sutras and Hatha Yoga Pradipika. My second series, Yoga Beyond the Poses: The Ultimate Beginner's Guide to Yoga, covers one yoga topic at a time and is extra easy to read with larger text. For those who find it challenging to read extensive books and want a good and broad overview of the subject quickly. Both series are also available as audiobooks.

Teaching Yoga and Meditation Beyond the Poses
– A unique and practical workbook for aspiring yoga teachers who want to teach yoga and meditation beyond the poses.

Teaching Yoga and Meditation Beyond the Poses is a unique and essential resource for new and experienced teachers and a guide for all yoga students interested in refining their skills and knowledge. Teaching Yoga and Meditation is also ideal as a core textbook in yoga teacher training programs.

The book covers fundamental yoga philosophy and history topics, including a historical presentation of classical yoga literature: Yoga Sutras of Patanjali, Bhagavad Gita, etc. Each of the seven major styles of yoga is described, from Hatha yoga, Raja yoga, Tantra yoga, Bhakti yoga, and Kundalini yoga, to knowledge about the chakras, Ayurveda and magic mantras and yantras. The book provides extensive support and tools for teaching integrated and classical yoga (asanas), breathing techniques (pranayama), deep relaxation (Yoga Nidra), and meditation (Ajapa Japa). The book is divided into eight modules with associated knowledge tests and complete yoga and meditation classes.

https://rb.gy/9s6edj

SIGN UP FOR A UNIQUE & FREE CHAIR YOGA CLASS WITH SHREYANANDA NATHA!

DO YOU WANT TO QUICKLY AND EFFECTIVELY LOSE WEIGHT? BECOME MORE FLEXIBLE? IMPROVE YOUR BALANCE? OR FIND PEACE IN LIFE AND RID YOURSELF OF STRESS? NOW YOU HAVE THE CHANCE!

SANKALPA YOGA *IS CLASSICAL YOGA & MEDITATION FOR CHAIRS CREATED BY BEST-SELLING AUTHOR AND YOGA MASTER SHREYANANDA NATHA. IT INCLUDES UNIQUE SERIES OF CHAIR YOGA THAT CAN CHANGE YOUR LIFE HERE AND NOW:*

* **CHAIR YOGA FOR BETTER BALANCE**
* **CHAIR YOGA FOR SOFTER JOINTS**
* **CHAIR YOGA FOR INCREASED STRENGTH**
* **CHAIR YOGA FOR GREATER FLEXIBILITY**
* **CHAIR YOGA FOR IMPROVED FITNESS**
* **CHAIR YOGA FOR WEIGHT LOSS**
* **RELAXATION & MEDITATION**

DURING THE TRIAL CLASS, YOU'LL HAVE THE OPPORTUNITY TO EXPERIENCE WHICH PROGRAM MIGHT SUIT YOU AND THE DEEP-ROOTED EFFECTS OF GENUINE CLASSICAL CHAIR

YOGA AND MEDITATION. THE CLASS IS LED BY SHREYANAN-
DA NATHA (MATTIAS), AND YOU'LL RECEIVE AN INVITATION
TO THE CLASS SENT VIA VIDEO LINK.

SIGN UP AT THE LINK:

https://shorturl.at/pxRTW

OR SCAN THE QR CODE:

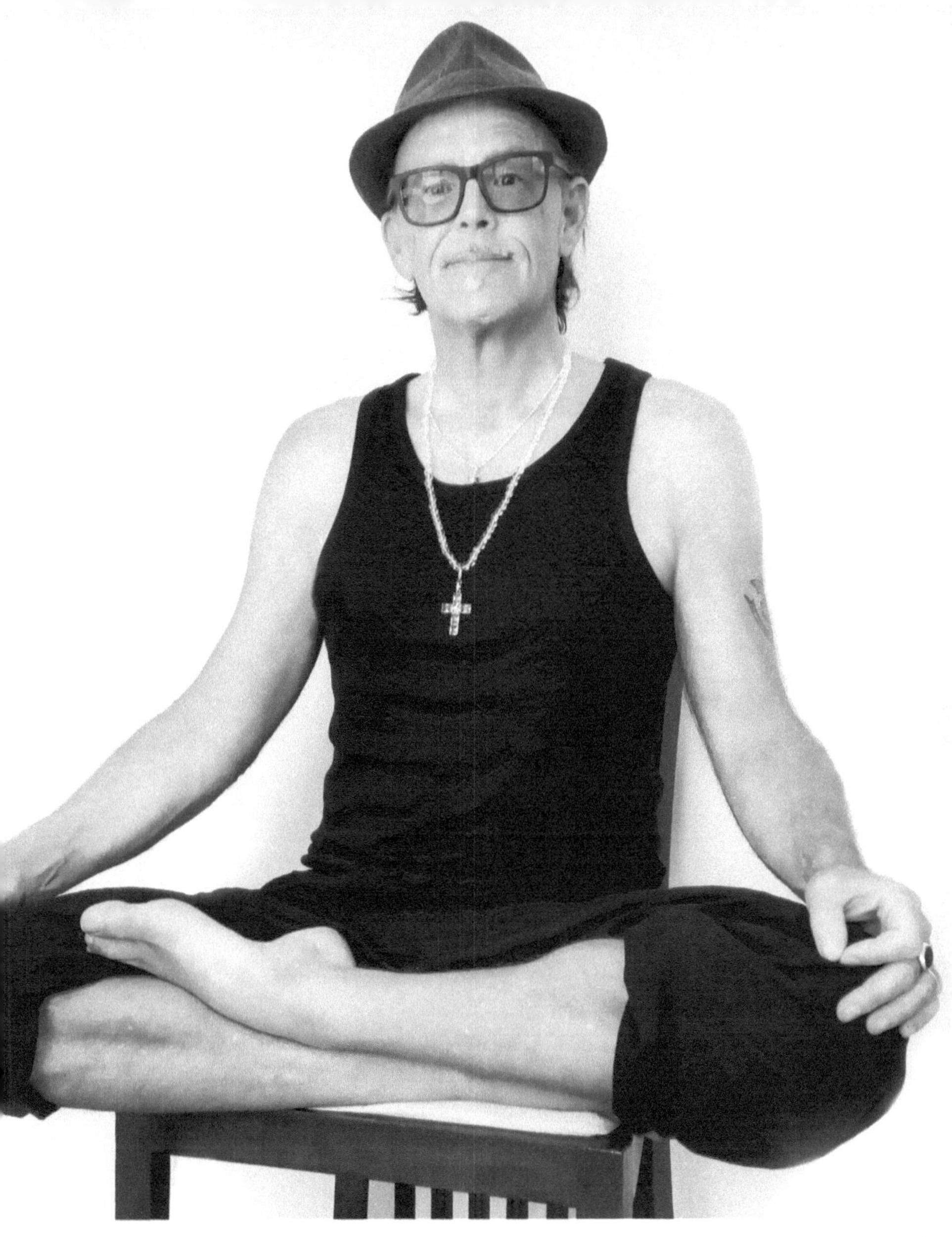

Namo Narayan!

Shreyananda Natha (Mattias)

www.ingramcontent.com/pod-product-compliance
Lightning Source LLC
LaVergne TN
LVHW051516170726
843492LV00002B/963